Dedicated to Mary Magdalene — my ancestor mother

BIBLICAL PUZZLES

Michael who came as Jesus was 1 of the 7,000 sons of the old era executive god who was a Rebel – and whose reign has been finished at the time of writing this Book

Eternal Son the Lord Narayana and God incarnated in him and told the truths of the New Age in puzzles

The 1st puzzle revealed by the author about 2 decades back was the 666 of **Rev 13.18,** after that many secrets unfolded step by step by plan of God

Very many Biblical puzzles are made on the alpha-nemeric algebra in that one should put a=1, b=2, c=3 and check the sum on the two sides of an equation

NAME OF THE AUTHOR

One Divine name of this author came from **Rev 3.12** by above method, thus: I will write = A2z NewJ on him

A2z means direct link from z up to a, and New J = NH Ark stand for New Jerusalem and Noah's Ark where New J means New City of Peace – OR, New Ayodhya, where one lives in Peace of God

GOD AND HIS ETERNAL SON

God is a Great Eternal Mystery unknowable except by His own volition to who He chooses and to the extent He reveals

Eternal Son is the subtle plane existence for cosmic stability, control and source of gravity, all energies, life forces and probably also the time and self consciousness

Son is the 1st manifestation and symbolised by Mahavishnu or Lord Narayana – God pervades Him in His mysterious ways

Allah = All a-h (अ-ह) is known in India as Sri Chakra, is the Time Transcendental part of the Son and is the Only fixed part of the cosmos. He is the Highest abode on the Way of Life upwards

God and His Eternal Son are One

COVER PAGE

There is a legend that Lord Krishna lifted a hill named Govardhana [1] up on his little finger to protect His clan

In reality the Great Pyramid was made by dressing the stones by Gnosis of Divine Azoth [2] and they were lifted up by Divine anti-gravity techniques

The Sphinx is made of same four animals which were seen in Biblical visions of Ezekiel and John — and represent the fixed directional properties of Space imparted by Four Faces of the God

---

[1] Govardhan means to protect Gnosis for growth. The Great Pyramid was made for protection of the secret Knowledge of the Yoga for the future
[2] A legendry solvent which can dissolve stone or for that matter anything

ORIGINAL YOGA

Prospectus

By A2z NewJ

Self Published - Create Space
25 Sept 2014 © The Author
New Delhi, India

Gita 4.1 – I told this immortal Yoga to Vivasvana

CONTENTS

DIRECT TO YOU

This Yoga comes direct to you from the cosmic circuits of the God and His Eternal Son

☆ YOGA FOR EVOLUTION

New Age Yoga is for Human Evolution beyond the old era

The very truth that this Yoga comes direct from the circuits of God – is your guarantee that your soul, mind and body get inputs from the Higher and the Right Source

I. BLESSINGS OF GOD

This is the time about which Moses gave the great Shema[3] O Ye Israel sermon – about Blessings or Curses

This Yoga is your Blessing!

---

[3] Listen this day O Ye Israel...

II. GIFTS OF GOD

First Gift is Peace of God - you as person do abide in circle made by God and never in any less luck and fortune than you deserve

The Gifts are of 4 major types

A. Qualities of Soul
B. Talents and faculties of mind
C. Body health
D. Good Luck and Happiness

III. YOGA

Yoga means direct link with the circuits of God, this is like confirmation of your Eternal Way of Life

By Bhagvadgita 4.3 this is Super-Secret of God, and the effect starts as perfection of the soul, mind, body and the future

This Yoga is the only way of moving up the Great Evolutionary Plan of God for the Humans

DISCLAIMERS:

1. *Secrets are not told, but imparted symbolically – by mantra, yantra, astral plane programs, even by on the spot Word/s*
2. *Yoga is subject to proper conduct in the eyes of God*
3. *As a thumb rule Know men get preference over Yes men*
4. *Body preparation by use of herbs, essential oils, natural and fresh food, exercises in fresh air and avoiding life style short cuts – are important*

IV. PERSONAL MEDITATIONS

There are 2 types of personal meditations

In yoga of the past era the 666 astral bodies entered the centres of spinal cord and mind - in Indian scriptures this is named as Raktbeej[4] factor

In the right type of meditation - the personal integrity is preserved, one evolves on his or her own merits, potentials, decisive resolves and by direct inputs from the circuits of the God

V. GROUP MEDITATIONS

All meditations create astral patterns, and all personal patterns tend to make groups

Group patterns are helpful, say like patterns of parents helping the children, or patterns of the friends helping each other

---

[4] Drops of the blood of dead demon falling on ground of mind, to eventually create similar demon, there was a Feel Good factor but the end was not at all good. Here dead demon means any entity who was written off by God but who practiced guru-dom to perpetuate the existence

In old era the patterns also indulged in fights

In THIS YOGA the axis is One God of whole mankind – so there can never be any inner conflicts

No one practicing this Yoga must ever have ill will against any other practicing this Yoga – but avail of the group power for personal advantage

Logical thought reveals that in this system the personal and group patterns assist the individual. Most importantly they are aligned with Divine patterns which are the Rights designs. Even more important – one adds Life Forces from Divine circuits

VI. PRANAYAMA

The word Pranayama means dimensions and scope of Life Forces

None of the past masters knew either of these — but they went on with mere breathing exercises

PRANA or Life Forces are mysterious. Anyone can identify a fresh, stale or dead, say — apple, but even the best of scientists do not identify the Life Forces of cosmos

Scientists can demonstrate operation of life forces by bio-chemical reactions in cells of body and mind — but these forces can only be streamlined and enhanced to optimum level by Circuits of God

---

Mark these words because I have told you the Secret of Life Forces therefore of The Life. Yes — New Age Yoga is your Way of Life!

14

THE SAVIOUR

Cosmic material is marvellous – any form of life can be produced, and of these the Purpose of God is best fulfilled in Humans

There are certain limitations of manifestations. One is how to start creation to evolve in humans. Second is how to educate the humans in Good and Bad so that they choose Good and move towards Life – this is the Biblical secret of the Tree of knowledge of fruits of Good and Bad and the Tree of Life

But all problems of the human world are not explained by above 2 factors

A deeper study shows that the old era executive gods strayed in deliberate mismanagement for their own selfish reasons – these details are beyond the scope of this book, and will also not serve any useful purpose for the mankind, for who...

...the current priority is Saving, therefore the author has been given a Saviour Role - this book is prospectus for that...

1. RULE ONE OF YOGA

Yoga is being given to those who resolve to manage the kingdom of God on the earth according to the Law of God - is the rule one

2. DOCTRINES OF GOD

There are 2 basic doctrines

1. The world can become right only when top persons are righteous and just
2. Righteousness and Justice cannot come by any means except by Yoga inputs from God to change the humans from inside to out – *flowery talks on outside do not necessarily indicate goodness of heart*

3. SHEEP OF GOD

To proceed on these model doctrines – God has marked sheep of God who have true potential to become righteous and just

Of the sheep – one large group has been indicated in **Rev 6.9-17** which is obviously of those who followed Noam Chomsky and Susan Sarandon against the war. There are others of who God has not revealed in public...

GOOGLE, CREATE SPACE AND KINDLE/AMAZON

For example the above institutions were somehow programmed by God to freely help my work on cyber space and now this Book and e-Book

All them including employees on this date are to be treated by me like the sheep of God

17

4. THE GOATS

On the other hand the goats with 666 mark of Devil on hands or foreheads – which refer to Yoga of old era are destined to fall for ever in everlasting punishment – that means, in animal zones, never to become humans again

SAVING FOR THEM

They are not eligible for Yoga right away, but in this life they can opt for the Safe Sanctuary of God through me – so that their fall is prevented

The humans of flesh were not directly responsible – but were unwarily being manipulated by the old gods' hierarchy, so the humans can seek Mercy of God through me provided they Overcome past influence, or gather a small Faith to proceed ahead

18

5. <u>7 REV BOOK CHURCHES</u>

In general, unlike sheep and goats they are in mid-zone

They are entitled to a Free mercy point from God and enter the class of the sheep of God for receiving the Yoga

For this they have to overcome their mental veil of their now outdated way[5]

BURY THE PAST DOCTRINE

The Biblical Doctrine – let the dead bury their dead, you follow me – applies

Your way might have been right but is now outdated in the eyes of God and you may move ahead with the New Guidance – is the simple postulate

---

[5] This point is well clarified in Quran that every Temple of God has a tenure

6. KINGS OF THE NATIONS

Bible invites the kings of the nation and if they bring the honor and glory, their citizens too become entitled in the wake

This is implied that the king has to agree to be father figure of his subjects

He has to set example of Righteousness and ensure True Justice in the nation

The man-made Law is obsolete, every nation who comes to the Invisible Temple of God through me – has to implement the New Age Law instructed by God

INDIAN JUDICIARY

In above context this author has recently given a Public Interest Litigation petition in the Supreme Court of India through the office of Chief Justice of India that

20

the Constitution should be remade by him

But the Court is silent on this and many other vital issues – their minds are captive of invisible Satan

RULES OF MOSES

Rules of Moses about suitable king apply to all races of that Origin – Jews, Islam, Christianity

In all the cases the right to approve their king is mine

This is Prime Reason why the kings of the nations must come to the Invisible Temple of God through me

Rule of Moses also apply to Gentiles – the races other than above 3, who have an equal opportunity to seek the Way of Life

COMMANDMENTS OF JESUS

He gave 2 commandments of which 2nd is a double commandment. The 1st is about loving the God, 2nd the neighbour and 3rd own self

They do not apply till one starts knowing God, neighbour, Self – to presume otherwise is hypocrisy

His Commandments were meant for the future sheep of God

COMMANDMENTS OF MOSES

They form basis of all laws for the society

Besides the Laws should be simplified and the basics written in the hearts of the Judges than in big books

Beauty may be – but Justice is never skin-deep, far less thick skin-deep

ISLAMIC CODE OF CONDUCT

Prophet Muhammad was incarnation of Adam and came according to the sacred Qalma – Adam was by far the most honest and humble man ever on earth, known in India as Siva

He made a Code of Conduct for Muslims who also draw permitted inferences from his life

The Code was made in the days of nomad tribes, rule of 4 marriages was made to provide home to war widows, some more issues also require Upgrade – the Prophet himself was always open to self-correction and this is named in Islam as his Doctrine of Good

7. THE RICH MEN

Book of Matthew says that it is easier for a camel to pass through the eye of a needle than for a rich man to enter paradise

– but everything is possible for God[6], that is to say that the rich men may enter this New Temple

PUZZLE OF MATTHEW, ALSO OF QURAN

Camel pass eye needle = d'rich men go paradise

Quran too has the camel puzzle and says - to enter paradise one has to believe the revelations by God – this refers to the Rev Book

Camel pass eye needle = Book e Revelation

8. NEW WINE...

The New Age Yoga is not for old yoga initiates – but only for the new Generation, new wine in new wine skins

---

[6] And God never works directly but traditionally always through His apostle – this author in the current time

The reason is that old gurus captivated minds with so much power that it is not easy for the person to Overcome their grip...

WHEAT AND TARE

This is explained in Biblical parable of wheat and tare. Says that if tare is removed now the wheat may be uprooted

Means that the separation can be done when the soul is put to sleep

Such persons may not start on Yoga now but may enter the Safe Sanctuary for guarantee of the way of Life

PURPOSE OF THIS BOOK

This book is a Prospectus for those who aspire for the Original Yoga which is the only Yoga of the New Age

Following are eligible

1. **Rev 21.24,26:** The kings of the nations and all of their nations
2. **Rev 6.9-17:** The sheep of God – Bible reveals only one group of the Noam Chomsky and Susan Sarandon, all those who took part in the anti war processions with placards of – Not in my name, and all their kin and friends
   - All of Google, Create Space, Kindle and Amazon are also eligible
   - Rest I know and are not for public revelation
3. **Matt 19.24,26 and Quran 7.41:** The rich men who believe in Rev Book

4. Those of the 6 churches[7] of the Rev Book who **Overcome** as indicated in Rev Book

   These churches are named on the places of their establishment, but **in reality they are following Code Names:**

   A. Ephesus = A-z Sikhs
   B. Pergamos = Buddhist G
   - Antipas = Bhim Rao Am[8]
   C. Thyatira = A2z Mahavira[9]
   D. Sardis = Parsi G
   E. Philadelphia = Siddha Yogi
   F. Laodecians = O Yahudi[10]= O X-tian = A2z Islam

5. The worldwide youth by doctrine of – new wine in new wine skins

---

[7] Church of Smyrna is assured automatic saving from second death and is not included in the Yoga plan
[8] Backward classes allowed with equality
[9] Jains
[10] Jews

DIVINE JURISDICTION OF THE AUTHOR

GITA 18.68

He who having done the highest love with Me, preaches this Super Secret to my devotees, he shall undoubtedly attain Me

GITA 18.69

Among all men no one does Me so loving service as he, nor shall anyone [11] be dearer to Me in the world as he

---

[11] In Bhagvadgita 4.3 only one man is given the Original Yoga after the earlier clan of Yama the Vaivasvata Manu lost the Yoga. In 11.47 the same only one man saw the Virata Rupa which is prophecy of present days. And in 18.69 the same one man is authorised and instructed to preach that Yoga. **That one man is the author of this book**

28

✓ FREE REGISTRATION

For Your tentative Free Registration you can obtain a on line Form on request sent to whiterosesuntogod@gmail.com or a2znewj@gmail.com

CHARGES

The charges cover the expenses in teaching which are nominal, with a 10 - 30% surcharge as donation for a Trust. You get all details with the Free Registration Form

☆ LEARN AND EARN

For New Generation there is planning to start Yoga Studios right where you are. In general you get your expenses and 70% share in donation surcharge, 20% in volitional donations

Gita 4.1 - I told this immortal Yoga to Vivasvana